SECRETS
OF JOINT PAIN

DR. SHABEER.M.S

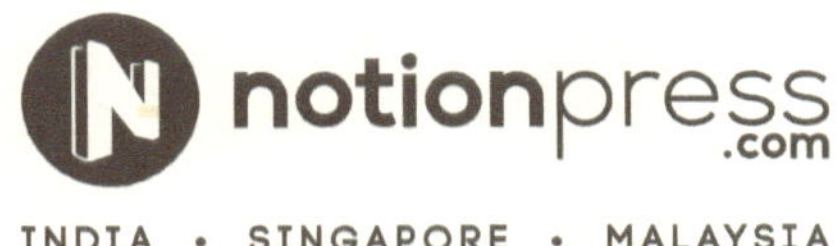

INDIA • SINGAPORE • MALAYSIA

ISBN 979-8-89233-397-9

1. **What are the causes of Joint Pain?** Broadly speaking, there are two causes of joint pain.

   First of all various types of injuries, bruises and fractures. The second category includes wear and tear, cancer and infection, etc. Or it can be divided into two such as traumatic and atraumatic.

   We can see many causes of joint pain depending on age.

   For example, hip joint diseases change with age. Common hip joint diseases in very young children are synovitis and congenital dislocation. Later diseases like Perthe's disease, tuberculosis and slip are seen. Osteoporosis and Osteoarthritis are the leading causes of joint pain in elderly people.

2. **What exactly are the causes of joint pain and how are they diagnosed?**

   It is very important to know the causes for diagnosis of arthritis. That too is diagnosed through two methods. First of all, direct examination of the patient or clinical examination. Secondly various lab tests. For example, tuberculosis is diagnosed through blood tests and sputum test.

3. Doctors are accused of doing more tests like scans unnecessarily. Is that correct?

Not right. It is true that some expensive tests are needed to detect certain diseases and to confirm the diagnosis. For examples, knee injuries such as meniscus injuries and anterior cruciate ligament injuries in young athletes can be detected by MRI. A scan can confirm the diagnosis. This is important because the treatment of both are different. The meniscus is the washer- like part between the knee bones. Its injuries are less severe than those of the anterior cruciate ligament. It is also easy to cure by keyhole surgery . At the same time, the arterior cruciate ligament injuries can only be repaired by ligament reconstruction. The cost will increase. This surgery cannot be done under local anaesthesia. In every disease like this, doctors advice scan and tests only for such essential things. To meet such expenditure the government should provide necessary financial assistance to them. There is a reason to say this. Compared to developed countries, only one tenth of the government's financial allocation for the health sector has been set aside for the medical sector from India's GDP. For this reason, doctors are often under the shadow of doubt. It affects the patient doctor relationship and the treatment results are badly affected

4. What are the treatment for joint pain?

Joint pain treatment will vary depending on the cause. That is depending on the diagnosis, the treatment will also change. For example, there are many causes of back pain. Some important reasons are Intervertebral disc prolapse, spondylosis, osteoporosis, spondylolysis, and akylosing spondylitis. Diagnosis should be done first. Methods like x-ray and scan can be adopted for it.

Now if the cause is osteoporosis, drugs can be given to increase the calcium level in the bones. A diet high in calcium is also important. If the cause is intervertebral disc herniation, treatment will vary depending on its severity. The severity is assessed through scanning. Disc herniation can be classified into four with the help of MRI scan.

A. Bulge

B. Protrusion

C. Extrusion

D. Sequestration

Pain relievers and lifestyle changes may be sufficient in the first grades. These include not lifting too much weight and bending. In the next stage, you can use belts, corsets etc. to give support to the back. In very advanced stages, the treatment methods are traction and epidural injection. At a stage that is not improved by these, the treatment is done by removing this disc through surgery.

5. Many people suffer from back pain. Is it related to joint pain?

That is a good question.

This is the complaint of many patients at ortho op in our hospital. They have back pain due to various causes. All the tests we do will be normal. But if you palpate that particular part of the pain, it will present as thickening in the hand that is deep in the muscles. Trigger point is a fibrotic nodule which is most likely the cause of such pain. Fibro myalgia is often treated with physical therapy, such as ultrasound therapy, or TENS therapy or injection in that area.

6. Do children get joint pains ?

There are some diseases seen especially in children. For example hip joint disorders mainly occur in pediatric age group are synovitis, dislocation (CDH) slip (SCFE) and Tuberculosis.

Perthe's disease patients show pain and limping. We diagnose the disease through various tests and give the necessary treatment.

The disease like synovitis can be cured by treatment with non weight bearing for a few days. But some surgeries will have to be done for hip dislocation depending on the age. Perthe's disease also sometimes requires surgery. Hip joint pain caused by tuberculosis will require tuberculosis treatment.

7. When is joint replacement surgery done?

Knee replacement surgery is now a very common treatment method. Knee or joint degeneration occurs mainly in the elderly. In the beginning, the pain is relieved by methods such as pain killers and exercise therapy, but as the severity of the disease increase, injection therapy and after that knee replacement surgery is performed.

8. Is knee replacement surgery successful?

Of course.

Total knee replacement is a surgical procedure in which the degenerated knee join is resected to the exact size with the help of a jig- like device, and then a metallic prosthesis of the same size is attached with the help of bone cement.

9. When do knee replacement patient start walking?

The patient is ambulated with the help of a walker within three days after the operation. This is after ensuring that the joint is secured in the correct position. With proper rehabilitative treatment, the patient can walk independently within two weeks.

10. What is the difference between rheumatoid arthritis and other joint diseases?

Osteo arthritis is what we denote commonly as wear and tear. It mainly affects knee and hip joint. But, rheumatoid arthritis is much more common in young population. Not only does it severely affect the joints of the hands, wrists, knees, neck, and feet, it also begin at a young age. Rheumatoid arthritis is more common in women.

11. How is rheumatoid arthritis diagnosed?

Diagnosis of rheumatoid arthritis requires routine clinical examination along with some special blood tests. ESR and rheumatoid factor are useful in this regard.

12. How is rheumatoid arthritis treated ?

In addition to regular pain relievers, there are disease - modifying anti- rheumatic drugs (DMARD). There are drugs like chloroquine, immune therapy is now emerged as an innovative treatment option. But it is very expensive.

13. Is it correct to say that there is a difference between men and women in joint pain?

That's right.

Rheumatoid arthritis is more common in women while disease like ankylosing spondylitis is quite different from that of rheumatoid arthritis as ankylosing spondylitis is common in men.

14. Is there a relationship between life style and joint pain?

Of course.

Arthritis pain varies according to the activities that each person does on a daily basis. For example, some people experience pain in the elbow joint. This condition, called tennis elbow, is treated with painkillers, injections, and tennis elbow straps.

But some people have pain in the wrist joint. This disease is caused by thickening of two muscle tendons in the hand. Then the patient can be treated by releasing the thick part through a small surgery. This disease is called Dequervain's tenosynovitis.

Both tennis elbow and Dequervain's disease fall into the category of repetitive strain injuries.

Another common disease is trigger finger. This is caused by thickening of the ring of muscle fibers leading to locking of the finger. Its release requires surgery. Many patients are struggling with these three conditions. It can be cured by simple surgeries.

Another disease that can be mentioned among these is carpal tunnel syndrome. The reason is the compression of the median nerve. This is due to narrowing of the carpal tunnel. That disease also requires a release surgery by which, the pain, numbness and weakness that have been disturbing the patient for a long time will be removed.

15. Is there a connection between osteoporosis and joint pain?

Of course.

Osteoporosis or bone loss is the loss of calcium in the bones. We know that all joints are made up of bones. Because of this, bone loss can cause joint pain. Bone mineral density is a measure used to diagnose osteoporosis. With the help of the BMD severity of the disease is divided into mild, moderate and severe and appropriate drugs are given. This is important because people with very low bone mineral density are more prone to fracture and is called the fragility fracture. Fractures of the wrist, hip and spine occur in elderly women with relatively minor falls. This is very common.

Especially in the present time, the elderly are living alone in their homes. Children may have gone abroad for work or study or even if they are at home, you will not see anyone at home during the day. Many people fall inside the house due to defective vision, dizziness, blood pressure changes, blood sugar changes etc. Thus patients with such fractures in old age will become a social problem and the government needs to intervene so that old men and women will not lead such a lonely life.

16. Is there any way to avoid such fractures?

Of course,

I mentioned that joint pain comes with osteoporosis. Then assuming that people with bone pain may have bone loss or osteoporosis, if they strengthen their bones through treatment, they can prevent colles fracture or wrist facture, hip fractures, and spine fracture that come in old age to some extend. More over, falls in the elderly need to be prevented. For that, defective vision, diabetes, high blood pressure and other diseases should be detected and controlled through regular comprehensive check-up. In addition to this, there is a need for social interventions to avoid loneliness and insecurity in the elderly.

17. Are ayurvedic treatments and acupuncture relevant for arthritis ?

That is a good question.

We know painkillers are primarily taken for arthritis. In physiology a lesson learned in the early years of MBBS is the gate control theory of pain. Based on that, methods like acupuncture, acupressure and ayurveda are good to some extend to reduce pain. Similarly heat therapy or thermal treatment and cryotherapy or cold treatment used in the physical medicine branch of modern medicine. TENS, SWD (Short Wave Diathermy) and contrast bath also relieves pain according to gate control theory.

But treating the root cause of the pain is different. For example, if you give pain killer injection for sprained shoulder pain will be removed. But the injury by that trauma will not heel. Pain of arthritis due to wear and tear can be relieved by methods such as massage therapy and heat therapy. But the damage of the worn out joints will not change. It is the same with other joint diseases such as meniscus injuries, anterior cruciate ligament injuries, spinal diseases such as disc prolaps etc. This is a matter that needs to be understood very clearly. Because this is a topic that causes a lot of confusion among the common people.

18. Is it true to say that if uric acid increases joint pain will occur ?

That's right.

Uric acid is a chemical commonly found in our body. Uric acid is produced as part of metabolic processes when eating more meat. When its quantity increases, it turns into crystal form and deposit inside the joints. It is a disease that causes intense pain and the disease can be diagnosed by testing the uric acid in the blood. Uric acid levels can be reduced with medicines like zyloric and feburic acid. The prevention of this disease is to avoid foods containing the chemical purine.

19. What are the cause of shoulder joint pain?

Every day many patients come to OP with shoulder pain. Shoulder pain can have many causes. Periarthritis is a common condition in people with diabetes and high cholesterol. The immobility caused by periarthritis can be reversed through physiotherapy and drug treatment. This is a disease that is very difficult for the patients. People with this condition have difficulty in dressing themselves. They are not able to move arm behind the body and above the head.

Another condition is rotator cuff injuries. The rotator cuff is the muscle group that covers the shoulder joint and helps in its movement. MRI scan is taken to know the exact injuries. Depending on the nature of the injury, at least some patients may Benefit from arthroscopic surgery.

Other diseases like bicipital tendinitis, shoulder hand syndrome and impingement disease can also cause pain in shoulder joint.

20. Some children are born with curved feet. Is it joint related ?

Good question.

Many children are born with clubfoot or CTEV, this disease is caused by abnormal alignment of the joints of the foot. It is known as congenital talipes equinovarus. It means that the foot is bent inwards and stuck downwards. Treatment with plaster of paris cast is effective. This treatment is known as the ponseti technique, which aims to correct such foot deformities.

21. What are the causes of joint pain in children?

Os good schlatter's disease is a disease causing pain in the knee. Pain killers and plaster of paris slabs are good for its treatment. Also some of the other joint diseases such as madelung disease in the wrist, radio ulnar synostosis in the elbow and sprengel shoulder in the shoulder joint are seen in children. These too can be accurately diagnosed and treated through examinations such as x-rays and scans.

Another birth defect is known as Erb's palsy. Erb's palsy is a hand disability caused by the entrapment of the nerves to the hand due to complications during child birth. Physiotherapy and brace treatment are also beneficial for this. A brace called aeroplane splint is helpful for this.

22. How is carpal tunnel syndrome diagnosed?

Diagnosis is mainly through clinical and other tests. Clinically the patient is subjected to two tests. First of all, it is suggested to do Phalen's test or to fold the patient's hands to the inside and keep them for one minute. Following this, the patient shows symptoms of pain, swelling and numbness.

Another test is called provocation test. When the elbow is extended and the wrist is folded to 60 degrees, as mentioned earlier if pain, numbness and tingling are seen, it can be assumed that there is carpal tunnel syndrome.

Another test is the nerve conduction test. Through this, the severity of compression of the median nerve passing through the carpal tunnel can be understood.

23. When is knee replacement required in patients with knee pain?

Clinical examination and x-rays are used to determine the need for surgery in patients with knee pain. While taking x-rays, the main thing is to look for how much is the gap between the bones of the knee has disappeared and if there is more swelling, it can be osteophyte caused by wear and tear on the knee. And knee stiffness occurs in old age. If all these are found, the patient will be advised for surgery.

24. Is there a day for osteoporosis like World Diabetes Day?

Of course, world **osteoporosis** day is celebrated every October. And October 20 is world osteoporosis day. This awareness campaign started from 1998 in a very effective manner. Each year focuses on a theme and this day celebrated. Osteoporosis commonly occurs in women over 40 years of age due to a decrease in calcium levels in the bones.

25. Does cancer cause joint pain?

Of course,

Cancer is mainly classified as primary and secondary. Example of primary tumor in bones is osteosarcoma.

But secondary is said to be a stage of cancer that is primarily in the thyroid, intestine and kidney and the patients will complain pain to the bones. When it comes as metastasis to the bones, the patient feel pain and swelling. If you look at bone tumors, there are two categories, benign and malignant.

Malignant is a more aggressive tumor. Benign tumors are divided into three categories according to the Enneking classification: latent, active and locally aggressive. An example of a latent is non-ossifying fibroma. It sometimes gets better on its own. Aneurysmal bone cyst comes in the active group. This tumour, becomes big, but will not go beyond a certain limit. But in the third, malignant tumours will grow beyond limits.

Gct or giant cell tumor is mainly seen in knee and wrist. At first it is felt as pain and after a while the patient will present with fracture.

Malignant tumors are further classified according to their source as osteosarcoma, chondrosarcoma, malignant Gct and ewing's sarcoma.

Fibrosarcoma, chordoma etc. are also of malignant group.

26. What are the diseases that require knee replacement surgery?

Mainly two.

i. Osteoarthritis

ii. Rheumatoid arthritis

27. Is there age and gender variation for arthritis?

80 percent will be more than 75 years old. There is no difference between men and women till the age of 55. But after 55 this disease is more in women.

28. Which patients require knee replacement?

Quality of life can be very poor due to knee pain. A women or a man suffering from the disease may have to have knee replacement when the disease interferes with their daily personal life or social life.

The next reason is constant pain every day. Knee replacement is also often required to restore normal function of the knee.

If the x-ray examination shows serious damage to the knee joint, its an indication for knee replacement surgery.

29. It has been said that surgery does not help after one stage. Is it right?

- Surgery is difficult when the knee pain is there for a long time and the movement is very much reduced.

- Similarly, if the deformity is beyond a certain limit, knee replacement surgery is difficult.

- Knee replacement is difficult in the condition called contracture.

- Surgery is difficult if knee instability is there.

- Muscle wasting is a difficult condition.

30. What should be considered before knee replacement surgery? Or any precautions to be taken before knee replacement surgery?

The patient needs to undergo preoperative tests. Before the surgery, tests like diabetes, thyroid gland disease, cholesterol level in the blood are done and all of them should be checked so that the surgery does not threaten the life of the patient. If necessary, the opinion of other specialist doctors should be sought in this regard. A qualified anaesthesiologist can give clearance if all tests are within normal limits and the patient is considered as fit for anaesthesia. After that the decision for surgery can be confirmed.

31. Briefly describe knee replacement surgery?

Of Course.

Many patients react with a little fear when they hear about knee replacement.

True, knee replacement surgery is a surgery with lot of technical aspects. However, there is no need to look too scared. It is a very successful surgery if adequate precautions are taken and surgical skill is assured

If we want to know how to do knee replacement, we have to understand the structure of our knee joint briefly.

The knee is made up of the femur at the top of the leg, the tip of the upper tibia where it joins the femurs, and the patella in front of these two bones.

In addition to these bones, there are also some parts that contribute to the stability of the knee. They are important in knee surgery or replacement surgery.

The two type of meniscus in the inner part, the ligaments that connect the bones are two cruciate ligaments and two collateral ligaments.

After surgery, even in some patients, there is a disease called deep vein thrombosis or DVT. This is mainly due to consequence of not doing dorsiflexion exercises or not moving the feet exactly as prescribed by the doctor after the surgery. This is something that the patient and caregivers should be very careful about.

Another thing is that along with precise surgery, prosthesis of good quality material, and meticulous planning is equally important.

Another thing is infection. After the surgery, the patient's hygiene, bowel and bladder care are the things that should be taken care of. If these are not done under proper supervision, there is a risk of infection at the surgical site. Stitches are usually removed within two weeks of knee replacement surgery. Until then, it is a matter of great attention.

Third is post- operative rehabilitation treatment including rehabilitation physiotherapy, muscle strengthening, etc. The patient should be able to walk better without pain than before surgery. For this, the co-operation and vigilance of the patient, accompanying relatives and caregivers is very important.

Brief description of the steps in knee replacement surgery.

- The distal end of the femur should be precisely cut and fixed.

- The leg, the tibia, should also be prepared by cutting off the upper part.

- Preparation of patella.

All these things are done with proper technical assistance. Appropriate machine, power saws, jigs, nails or pins for measuring accuracy, and alignment rods all together make a knee replacement surgery, a procedure which requires lot of skills. This surgery is done only with adequate technical support.

No matter how complicated the surgery, if the accuracy is assured, it is a surgery that can be expected to be a complete success. The complete cooperation of the patient and relatives is also required.

32. Ok doctor, almost got an idea about the surgery. This is done for osteoarthritis knee. What kind of people does this happen to, or what are the risk factors for it?

Age is the first risk factor.

Our knees will naturally experience wear and tear after 50 or 60 years.

That is why obese people get this disease earlier. Another factor is that women are more prone to this disease. We know women have less muscle strength than men. Especially the quadriceps muscle in the thigh. Quadriceps is a muscle group composed of four muscles: vastus medialis, vastus intermedialis, rectus femoris and vastus lateralis.

Quadri means four.

Hence the name quadriceps. By excercising this muscle complex regularly and correctly, strengthening of muscle happens which can reduce the wear and tear to some extend. Some other factors are injuries, infections and persistent occupational trauma.

Infection can also lead to wear and tear. Another cause is rheumatoid arthritis.

33. What are the symptoms of wear and tear?

- Mainly pain
- Then difficulty in doing daily activities(loss of function)
- Stiffness
- Swelling
- Hearing of sound from the joint when joint is flexed.

34. What are the non- operative treatment?

The first thing is to make the patient aware about all the above mentioned things.

For example, obese people should be give instructions on how to reduce weight.

And if the patient needs an assistive device we can give a walking stick.

- Weight loss
- Physiotherapy
- Then drug treatment

35. What are drug treatments?

It is mainly pain killers.

Next are the drugs known as glucosamine. Then the medicine which can be injected into the joint.

It can be steroid or hyaluronic acid. It reduce the pain.

36. What are the causes of joint degeneration?

- Over weight
- Bad habits
- Strenuous work
- Jobs which require prolonged Standing (police, doctor, teacher etc...)
- Smoking
- Alcohol
- Excessive sports
- Old age
- Previous disease: Rheumatoid arthritis, Septic arthritis.
- Previous fracture and injuries

37. What is arthroscopy?

Arthroscopy is a means of viewing the inside of joints. Many patients with abdominal pain are treated through laparoscopy by general surgeon. That is laparoscopy which is an advanced technique for viewing the inside of the abdomen. Similarly, we in orthopaedic surgery, use arthroscopy to treat joints without making large skin incision. These innovative methods are now used in almost every speciality. In ENT, FESS is a sinus surgery done through endoscopy. In gynaecology it is called hysteroscopy. The word meaning of the word scopy is to see within. So we can say that arthroscopy means visualization of interior of joint.

38. Is this arthroscopy performed in all joints?

Mostly now it is done in knee and shoulder joint. Other joints such as hip and ankle can also be done.

39. Will you please explain the instruments used for arthroscopy?

That is a good question.

We often hear about arthroscopy or keyhole surgery. But due to the ignorance regarding its details, the common people still see it as extraordinary and are averse to such surgery. Knowing what an arthroscope is, can help alleviate this confusion to some extent.

An instrument called as arthroscope consists mainly of a tube-like component called trocar. It is with it an arthroscope, similar to a telescope, is inserted into the joint to view the joint. The eyepiece is at the outer end or outer tip of the scope. An electrical light bulb can also be found inside. Lens can also be seen behind this bulb. This lens magnifies the microscopic parts of the joint and shows it on the display monitor, This is another advantages of the arthroscope. We can see many pathologies or diseases that cannot be seen with the naked eye through arthroscopy. That is why arthroscopy is used to diagnose many diseases. Arthroscopy is prescribed for many patients and diagnose many conditions of joint as it is not as expensive as MRI scan. This is called diagnostic arthroscopy.

40. Can you elaborate on the arthroscope or the procedure?

Of course,

Arthroscope can only be done under anaesthesia with regional anesthesia or spinal anaesthesia as the initial step.

The area of the joint for arthroscopy is given anesthesia and small incision is made to pass the scope. It's too small like a space to pass a pen. This is called portal through which trocar is introduced. After drainage of the synovial fluid, which is accumulated in the joint, saline solution introduced into it and then trocar is introduced into the saline solution that has been prepared for swelling and the joint is swollen. There will also be a stop coke attached to the trocar so that each one is properly magnified and viewed on the monitor.

Then the scope is passed through the trocar and a detailed visual inspection of each part of the joint is done very systematically. For this, the arthroscopic surgeon should have some technical expertise. That is why doctors are willing to sacrifice their time for various trainings.

The main skills required are sweeping, pistoning, rotation and triangulation. Sweeping involves moving the scope sideways horizontally and vertically up and down to see the inside of joints.

The second skill is called pistoning. This is done by moving the inner tip of the scope a little further in and out to make the sight look a little better. We know. when the scope is brought closer to a part, the part is magnified and more subtle disease conditions can be seen. When taken out, the surrounding areas of the part are also seen more and field of vision will be more.

The next skill is called rotation. You can move the arthroscope in a 360 degree arc. This is important because the tip of the inside of the scope sits at 25-30 degrees, so that 360 degree rotation allows you to see more of the interior.

The most important skill required for an arthroscopic surgeon is triangulation. Triangulation is the skill of correcting, balancing or shaving a diseased joint detected by sweeping, pistoning and rotating movements of the scope inserted through the second portal and first portal. It requires lot of training. This is why at least some orthopaedic surgeons specialize as arthroscopic surgeons.

It is a current trend. It is called super specialization like spine surgeon and hand surgeon.

41. Knee pain is a very common problem people talk about. Can you clarify the structure of this knee joint?

It is a good question. To clearly understand the causes and solutions of knee pain, it is necessary to know the structure of knee joint. Because the knee is the joint that plays an important role in supporting the body weight, it has special characteristics.

First of all, the knee joint is formed by the femur, the tibia, fibula, and patella.

Next, the knee joint is called the compound synovial joint. The reason it is called compound is that two types of movement are possible. The first is the saddle type patello femoral joint which is similar to leather seat located on the race horse. Secondly, the movement of the femorotibial joint which is known as the hinge joint. This is similar to the movement of the door. The femorotibial joint is designed to flex approximately 90 degree.

The third feature of the knee is that it has a covering called the synovium. This is called synovial joint. This is important to know, because synovitis is a disease that affects this lining. Similarly, another disease is synovial chondromatosis. Some of this disease affects this covering. Disease like synovial TB also affect it. Such disease can be distinguished only by knowing that there is such a cover in the knee joint.

The fourth feature is that the knee joint is not like the hip joint. A ring of muscles around the hip joint protects it from certain injuries. But the knee joint is not like that. It is superficial and because of that there is more chance of injuries due to accidents, falls, etc.

The next characteristic is related to the stability of the knee joint. You can understand it by relating it to the hip joint. The hip joint or elbow has stability due to the specific shape of the bones. These joints are known as ball and socket. That is, as if a ball is placed in a socket - like cup. This is not the case for the knee. Below that, the upper part of the tibia is flat. But in the femur or thigh bone, there are two condyles like "w" letter, located on the top of the tibia. It is not a stable structure like the hip and elbow joints. Therefore, the bones are supported by two ligaments inside, two ligaments on the sides and the quadriceps muscles. This is also important. Because injuries to these can lead to problems for the knee joint.

Sixthly, the structure of the knee joint has many elements called bursae around the knee. Bursitis disease also present as knee pain and then inside the knee is a structure called the meniscus.

It can be injured in violent strain while playing various sports games like football. Another feature of knee joint is outward angulation called Valgus. It is 7 degree. It will be slightly more in women. This is very important in surgeries like knee replacement.

These are the things you need to know about the anatomy of the knee joint.

42. What are the causes of knee pain ?

There are different types of pain in the knee joint. The knee is a common joint that gets injured due to running or accident. This is called mechanical reasons.

Illness like swelling in many parts of the body around the knee are next. These are called inflammatory conditions. These include synovitis, bursitis, and tendonitis. Blood related disorders such as rheumatoid arthritis, haemophilia, and sickle cell disease can also cause knee pain.

Another common disease is osteoarthritis.

Fifthly, some cancers also cause knee pain. Finally knee pain is also referred as diffuse pain of some disease of the pelvis and spine.

43. Does knee pain occur only in the elderly or in all age groups?

Knee pain can occur at any age. But causes are different. For example the discoid lateral meniscus, osteochondritis dissecans, osgoodschlater's disease and dislocation patella are mostly seen in people under the age of 18.

Diseases that come next up to the age of forty are mainly rheumatoid arthritis, meniscus injuries, and chondromalacia patella.

Degenerative disorders usually appear after age 40, but if other medical conditions and injuries have gone untreated, wear-and-tear can occur earlier. This is called secondary osteoarthritis.

44. A normal x-ray or scan is recommended for knee pain. Before that, what things are sought from the patients?

A variety of causes of joint can be diagnosed by mainly knowing the symptoms from the patient's own words. Many people report the same symptoms in different ways. Understanding this and asking for accurate symptoms is very important and a basic step in diagnosis

For example, do you feel or hear a clicking sound without pain, or does the knee become locked and unable to bend? Or do you fall down due to weakness of your knees

After that the tests or clinical examination can be done to confirm our diagnosis.

45. What does the doctor mean by clinical examination?

Primarily the clinical examination is visual examination. Inspection of the shape of the knee joint, Alignment, walking pattern and whether the thigh muscles are atrophied or swollen.

Then other tests or palpation test are done. On palpation, the knee may be warm and swollen if infection is there.

Only after these detailed examination the decision for surgery can be made.

46. Will you please explain special tests ?

That is a very good question.

There are many special tests. As I said, due to the unique structure and anatomy of the knee joint, there are different tests for different disease conditions. That is why it is called the special test. I am referring to the need for patients to state their medical conditions in a very precise and clear manner as the busy Orthopaedic OP has time constraints to carry out all the tests in detail. This is what should be aimed at with such books. Without adequate awareness, the disease conditions cannot be properly diagnosed. For example, in our government hospitals, 200 to 300 or sometimes more patients are seen in the Orthopaedic Surgery OP every day.

For each patient, It is not practical to do all the clinical tests at the beginning. Because there are numerous special tests such as Steinman test, Macmurae, Apley's, Lac Man, Dreyer test, Clark test, Wilson test, Fauchet test, Q angle etc. Each one is for knowing the problems of each part of the knee joint. To examine each patient in detail requires at least half an hour per patient. This is not possible in hospitals with 250 and 300 OPs. Therefore, an accurate diagnosis can only be made if the patient cooperates with the doctor's initial questions and tests very actively.

Similarly, another thing to understand is that not all patients can be diagnosed with technology such as x-rays and scans.

47. What are the other problems besides knee pain?

Mainly tumors.

Then the stiff joint. Another problem is locking in which inability to extend the knee joint. A condition known as clicking is also there.

Various angulations are seen. If it is inward, it's called genu varum and if it's outwards it's called genu valgum.

48. The doctor said that tumors can come to the knee without pain. What are the reasons for that?

Apart from bony growths or exostosis, and some types of tumors, the causes of knee pain can be categorized into three.First, there is a build-up of fluid in the joint. This fluid may be from synovium, the lining of the joint. This is called synovial fluid, or it may be bleeding that accumulates inside the joint after an injury.

Otherwise, it may be due to some infection and pus formation.

The second is inflammation of the synovium or synovitis. Third is the hypertrophy of this synovium, or an increase in size due to infection, which occurs in rheumatoid arthritis and TB, which affects the joint.

49. From what has been said so far, it has been understood that knee swellings can be diseases ranging from malignant cancer to rheumatoid arthritis and tuberculosis. How do you recognize this disease from other diseases ?

The first step is to closely monitor the condition of the knee joint. In other words, it should be seen whether the swelling is within the synovial membrane of the joint. An experienced orthopedic surgeon will be able to understand that. If so, it may be synovial effusion, haemorrhage, pyarthrosis, rheumatoid arthritis, tuberculosis or any other disease within the joint. If the swelling is beyond the limits of joint, three possibilities are there.

1. Fracture

2. Tumour

3. Infection like septic arthritis or osteomyelitis

After this clinical examination, simple blood tests, x-rays and MRI scan(if necessory) often lead to an accurate diagnosis.

50. From what the doctor has said so far, isn't it that all tumors are not malignant cancer and other causes also present as swellings in the knee joints?

That's right.

And people should know this. Because many people get lot of fear when they see a swelling on the knee or anywhere else. They will continue their living with great fear. There is no need for it. But don't take it for granted. You need to see a doctor soon to find out if it could be any of the reasons I mentioned earlier. An experienced orthopaedic surgeon can arrive at an accurate diagnosis

I have one more thing to say at this point. Apart from cancer, it has been said that there are many reasons for pain on the knee and around it. Cystic swellings are another group of diseases that should be mentioned here. Need to know this. Because many patients are stressed by the fear of these types of swellings misunderstanding as malignant cancer. This is caused by the accumulation of serous fluid in various parts of the body called bursae around the knee. It is known by various names as Clergyman's Knee and House Maid's Knee depending on its position.

Clergyman's knee tend to come in people who pray on their knees in church. But as a housemaid, you sweep the floor at home by standing on bent knee. A disease that comes over the prepatellar bursa that comes to housemaids who stand on their knees is called housemaid's knee.

Similarly, tumors are found in the popliteal region, which is the back of the knee joint. One of them is known as Morant-Baker cyst. Not only this, there are many other diseases.

Pigmented Villonodular Synovitis, synovial hemangioma, radomyosarcoma etc. are some of them. Treatment for each is different and some conditions are severe. So whenever you see swelling anywhere, a specialist doctor should be consulted as soon as possible. Find out what it is. Get proper treatment.

51. Back pain is a very common problem. What are the most important reasons?

The first cause of back pain that we always hear about is disc problems, which are generally experienced as pain that radiates to the groin, buttocks, or shins. This pain usually spreads to only one part of the body. Bilateral pain is rarely seen. It also increases when you cough, sneeze, or do other strenuous activities. This pain is worse when bending forward but decreases when sitting. This pain starts in the midline. Or this pain starts from the middle of the spine. The next category of pain is caused by the muscles and ligaments. This is because of the hard work done without adequate preparation.

Moreover, the pain is felt on one side of the back.

The third cause of pain is due to stiffness or spasm. It is usually seen early in the morning. After a while the pain subsides. Pain in this area usually resolves within two weeks.

Next is the category of back pain known as sciatica. It is seen at the location of the sciatic nerve. Not only is leg and foot numbness associated with this, but also weakness in the thigh, leg, and foot. These patients, who exhibit gait variation, often have difficulty in bowel and bladder evacuation.

Although back pain can be caused by many reasons, the above are the most common causes.

52. People who are obese or overweight are more prone to back pain. Can you explain that?

People who are overweight are more prone to back pain. A factor in the Back Pain Risk Assessment Test is obesity. According to it, a score of 1 is given for 6-7 kg, but those who are 12/13 kg overweight are twice as likely to develop back pain as those in the first category.

53. Now overweight people are increasing everywhere. Can you explain a little more how it causes back pain?

of course, That's right.

Most of the people these days are doing sedentary jobs.

IT Profession and other office work are effortless jobs. As a result, they gain weight because they don't get enough physical activity to burn the calories they eat every day. The body weight limit is the weight according to the height of each person. For simple calculation, it is said that the required body weight of each person is 100 less than the height. For example, if a person's height is 150 cm, then his maximum permitted weight is 50 kg. If a person is 10% overweight, not only back pain, but also shortness of breath, fatigue, and indigestion begin. If a person has 20 kg more than he needs, he will feel like a person walking with a 20 kg bag of rice tied around his waist.

In such overweight people, there are differences in the shape of the body from normal. For example, the normal forward curve of the spine, or lordosis, is altered. Because of this, some vertebrae are stretched. Moreover, nerve compression occurs as a result of the narrowing of the foramina through which the nerves pass.

Apart from this there is wear and tear in the vertebral joints.

Back pain in pregnant women should be understood in this context

On top of this, the muscles around the spine in the back of those with a pot belly have unnecessary strain on them. As we can imagine, if we walk with some weight on the right hand, the body will balance to the left. Likewise for those with pot bellies, the body balances backwards

The muscles will become tight. This is to correct the imbalance in the body caused by excess fat. This is how excess weight can lead to back pain

54. How is overweight easily diagnosed in the general population?

About half of our excess fat is stored under our skin. So if you feel the skin with your thumb and index, you can feel obesity. The skin below the navel should be held like this. If you gain more than 2 cm, you are overweight. But in women it is estimated to be three centimeters.

55. OK. If one realizes that he is overweight using the above methods, what are the methods to reduce weight?

If you realize you are somehow overweight, the next goal should be to reduce it. It has two ways.

1. Calorie-restricted diet

2. Regular exercise

56. Can you explain what is calorie restricted diet ?

Before that both these methods i.e. controlling food and increasing exercise should be included in our daily routine. It's not so easy, because we are following a fixed routine for decades. It is never possible to change it overnight. First we have to prepare our mind for it. Let's take a look at the benefits of losing excess weight.

Diseases like sleep apnea, depression, and migraines are reduced if overweight is reduced, and the risk of diabetes, hypertension, and heart disease are reduced. Risk of metabolic syndrome, arthritis, peptic ulcer, and fatty liver are also reduced. It also reduces chance of Type 2 diabetes, polycystic ovarian disease (PCOD), gout, stress, urinary incontinence and hyper cholesterolemia.

After knowing this, you should prepare your mind for a change in routine. For this we should understand the relation between the food we eat and the energy we need for daily life

Let's imagine that if we eat 1800 calories a day and the 1600 calories we spend on our daily physical activity, we consume 200 calories extra food. If we eats 200 calories per day, we will gain 1 kg in 40 days which is equal to 7716 calories. If you eat 1000 calories more than your daily requirement per day, you will gain a kilo in a week

Next we need to monitor our food intake accurately. For this we need to understand what is BMI. BMI is calculated by dividing the body mass in kilograms by the square of the height in metres.

Or BMI = $\dfrac{\text{weight(Kg)}}{\text{Height x height (m}^2)}$

Depending on our body weight it is classified into several categories as follows

<18 5- Underweight

A healthy person has a BMI between 18.5 and 24.9

If it is between 25 and 29.9, it is considered overweight. Between 30 and 34.9, the stage is called obesity. Between 35 and 39.9 is stage II, while over 40 is stage III obesity.

Name	BMI	Date

With such a chart we can improve our weight controlling.

57. When back pain occurs, it is said that the disc is faulty. Is that the only cause of back pain?

It is not correct to say that all back pain is caused by a misaligned disc. Back pain is caused by muscle and ligament strain also. Bends in the spine can also cause pain. These are known as scoliosis and kyphosis. Spondylosis can also cause pain. This is a form of wear and tear. Facet joint injuries can also cause back pain.

Infections of the spine, tuberculosis, osteoporosis and tumors can also cause back pain.

58. Is there a connection between pot belly and back pain?

Of course

Abdominal muscles protect the spine in three ways. The abdominal muscles and iliopsoas attach to the hip bone from the lumbar vertebra of the spine. Due to the weakness of these muscles, the joints and other ligaments quickly degenerate in those who do heavy work.

Secondly, these muscles also resist the position of the postural droop.

The abdomen is arranged like a sack full of intestines and other organs, with the pelvis below, the spine behind, the dome-like diaphragm above, and the extra- abdominal muscles in front. Although the tubes and intestines within it vary in quantity, a common factor is that they contain 80-90% water. The elements inside the abdomen are not compressible or shrinkable. So when we inhale the diaphragm muscle expands downwards. As a result there is a push forward. When you inhale too deeply, the diaphragm descends further to make room for the inflated lungs, like an inflated football strapped to our stomach

The opposite happens when we cough. The football, which is imagined to be attached to the stomach, comes to the top and the unwanted particles are expelled by the air that is pushed out.

But when we lift a heavy object, the diaphragm and abdominal wall contract together. As a result, the football, which is thought to be strapped to the abdomen, will give stress to spine. It will also cause back pain in the future.

People with who do not have strong abdominal muscles, will results in back pain in the future.

While not having a flat abdomen was once a beauty symbol, today a flat abdomen can be considered an essential component for the biomechanical efficiency of a healthy body for the above reasons.

For this reason, it is important to keep a check on the belly and to do regular exercises to strengthen the muscles around the stomach.

59. This is a very good knowledge. Now, can you explain the exercises for strengthening the muscles around the abdomen?

Let's start with some simple exercises. Lie on a flat surface with both arms by your sides. Then bend your knees slightly to bring them closer to your chest and stretch your body forward as if you are propelling a rowing boat forward with your legs, and stretch your arms to touch your feet. Come back to the original lying position. Repeat this ten times. This exercise routine is done to strengthen the muscles around the abdomen.

Excercise that strengthen the muscles around the abdomen without special preparations while doing some other things in daily life help you live without back pain. Here, the abdomen is pulled inward to bring it closer to the spine behind the navel. This is helpful. It can be done while driving, watching TV, or standing in a queue at Super Market. A third exercise known as the trunk twist can also be done very simply. Sit on a flat surface with both legs extended forward. Hold both the palms together and hold them behind the neck. Then lean to the left side and try to twist so that the right elbow touches the left knee. Then reverse the same way and try to twist the other side or the right side so that the left elbow joint touches the right knee. Repeat it ten times.

If we do the first rowing exercise, the second pelvic tilt exercise, and the last one in the trunk twist method it will strengthen back. If we combine it with a proper diet to some extent, we can strengthen the abdominal muscles and protect the spine so that back pain does not occur.

By strengthening the abdominal muscles in this way, our body posture will improve.

60. Starting from the bottom of the head, from the neck to coccyx the place where we sit, there is spine. But what is the reason for back pain seen more common in lower spine ?

That's a good question.

There are some reasons behind this which are biomechanical factors of the spine. The base of the spine is a very vulnerable area in the bony chain from the neck to the coccyx. This is because it is the junction between the relatively immobile hips and the ever-moving spine. It is called Lumbo Sacral Junction.

Every activity of daily life puts a strain on this lumbar joint. For example, when we bend forward to put shoes, when we close the window, or when we suddenly turn around and reach for the phone when the phone rings, the lumbo sacral joint is stressed more and more.

In this case, you may remember when electrical wiring is done in our house, the electrician breaks small wires. Holding a player like device in one hand, the other part of the wire is moved up and down several times with his right hand to break the wire. Electricians can cut electrical wires using this method known as stress fatigue. Similar fatigue happens at the lumbo sacral junction at the base of our spine as well.

At lumbosacal joint, your sacral part like the tip of the wire held still by the electrician through the countless work of daily life, and the lumbar portion, like the tip of the wire moving forward and backward, forms a fatigue strain in that area. For those with weak hamstrings and abdominal muscles, this fatigue is tenfold. People who lead an unhealthy lifestyle usually experience lower back pain.

61. It is a new knowledge. Then without knowing it, we are causing problems to the spine in many ways. Great to know. Now we can pay attention.

No, I didn't mean to keep your spine still, thinking that. Here are some survival tips so that we don't get overwhelmed by such daily activities in our life, have come into the body as a result of the process of evolution. One of them is thoracolumbar fascia

The story of the electrician is repeated once again. The thoracolumbar fascia acts as a covering for the spine, providing insulation similar to plastic or rubber insulation or flex that resists breakage of the electrically conductive wire by repeatedly folding it back and forth.

At the lumbosacral junction where most strain come, part of this fascia is considered the thickest.

Like a safety harness or a belt used by people with back pain, this fascia goes up from backbone as shown in the image below.

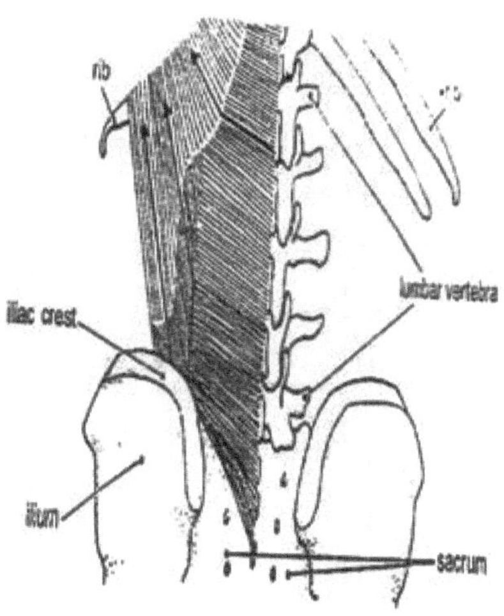

This thoracolumbar fascia protects the spine from the strain of bending and loading. The strength of this body part helps in this. This thoracolumbar muscle is formed in three layers, and below it attaches to the sacrum, the iliac crest of the pelvis, and the protruding spinous processes of the vertebrae known as the lumbar vertebrae. From there the fibers of this fascia extend upward and outward to join the three main muscles. Two of these are the abdominal muscles and the third is a strong latissimus dorsi muscle near the shoulder joint.

This sheath is superior to flex made of rubber or plastic placed around electrical conductors. It means that tension or pressure can be increased or decreased in various ways.

For example, doing things that require a lot of flexibility can reduce the strain on the latissimus dorsi and abdominal muscles and the thoracolumbar fascia. On the contrary, those who do very strenuous work are able to strengthen the spine enough to do heavy work with their strength.

It also has some practical relevance. One of them can strengthen the lower back by strengthening the abdominal muscles and the lattisimus dorsi muscle.

62. Correct. Exercise methods to improve strength of abdominal muscles were discussed in the previous questions known as rowing, pelvic tilt, and trunk twist. Now it is good to know how the latissimus dorsi muscle can be strengthened through exercise. Will you please explain that?

That's right. Now don't you understand that the latissimus dorsi muscle should be strengthened along with the abdominal muscles to prevent back pain? The main function of this muscle is to bring the arms closer to the body. The chin up exercise routinely recommended by military and police recruits is often used to strengthen the latissimus dorsi.

A chin up is an exercise in which you hang on a strong metal bar, folding both arms and raising your chin to the metal bar. It is instructed to do this twelve times or until the muscles feel tired. But since it is a difficult form of exercise, it is recommended for young athletes and armed forces trainees.

Instead, another method is recommended for people with back pain and older patients. Place both palms on the hips and elbows should be placed outwards. Then press down and firmly. Back pain can be kept away to some extent by doing the pelvic tilt, roving, trunk twist exercises that strengthen the abdominal muscles mentioned earlier along with chin ups or pelvic press.

63. Are any other forms of exercise effective in preventing back pain?

Good question.

As important as strengthening muscles is flexibility in the movement of all joints. People with wear and tear on the joints and arthritis often experience cramps in the muscles at the back of the leg, known as hamstrings, and associated parts of the joints, such as the calf. Its weight distribution is not balanced when doing heavy and strenuous work. As a result, more strain will be there at Lumbosacral Junction. This can cause back pain.

Therefore, along with muscle strengthening exercises, it is good to do proper physiotherapy for parts such as hamstrings muscles to remove the tightness and facilitate mobility.

64. Can strengthening exercises and stretching exercises around the waist prevent back pain?

Not only that, it is good to pay attention to some other things as well. For example, to maintain the correct posture is to maintain a balanced position of the body whether one is standing, sitting or lying down. If you are a regular driver, the correct position of the driving seat in the car etc. is important. And the condition of the bed is also important. Even the constant use of ill- fitting footwear can cause back pain for many people. And some rare diseases can also cause back pain. It should be checked by a doctor. Apart from all these, people who work in certain professions are more prone to back pain. This is called work- related back pain. Also, things like stress can also cause back pain. There are several medical conditions known as psychosomatic disorders. Certain types of infections can also cause back pain. Bladder infections and other diseases causes back pain. Those who insist on avoiding back pain should also pay attention to the above mentioned reasons.

65. I understood the exercise treatments to prevent back pain. Can you clarify what is the correct posture?

One thing should be noted here. Exercise therapy is presented very simply. Exercises such as Rowing, Trunk Twist in detail have been explained in such a way that they can be easily implemented in everyday life. Some other exercises like chin up and pelvic press were also explained in a simple way like this.

People with weak muscles and joint stiffness are more likely to experience lower back pain. Back pain risk can be checked with very simple flexibility tests. For this, it is suggested to touch the toes without bending the knees. The flexibility of one's spine can be measured by the gap between the fingers and toes.

Decreased lumbar flexibility is a sign of persistent and recurring back pain. The importance of regular back exercise is explained in five ways as below.

1. To strengthen the accessory muscles of the waist thereby helping to act as a cushion protecting the spinal joints from various types of strain or stress.

2. Sitting or standing for long periods of time To get a relief for one who is doing all the work for long period of time, regular exercise helps.

3. Regular spinal exercises help to relieve muscle strain and tension.

4. Stretching exercises to maintain flexibility of spinal joints is useful

5. Function of Muscles such as tendons, ligaments, and ligaments are based on the strength of the spine. The strength of the bones in the spine can also be maintained through regular core exercises.

66. OK. So apart from the previous exercises, what other exercises are included in regular exercise?

The most important of these is the William exercise, which is known all over the world. There are six types of exercises.

1. The first is to strengthen the muscles around the abdomen. It is similar to rowing.

   First lie on a flat surface. Fold both hands to the chest and slightly bend the knees. Keep your head, neck and shoulders lifted forward. Do not change knee position. Then release the arms and place them on the front surface near the feet. Then bring back the head, shoulders, and hand to return to the original position. Do this 5 to 20 times depending on each person's health condition.

2. The second exercise is to strengthens the gluteus maximus muscle

   For this, as in the first exercise, lie on a flat surface with both hands on the stomach, slightly bent legs. Place both hands on the navel area to ensure that the lumbar spine does not rise up. Then strengthen the buttock muscles behind the hips. By this, the lower part of the pelvis (base) also hits the surface.

Repeat this 10 to 20 times.

3. The third is very important exercise. For this, lie on a flat surface with both hands on your knees and pull your knees towards your chest. This should be repeated ten times.

4. It should be done while sitting on a flat surface. Sit with both legs stretched forward.

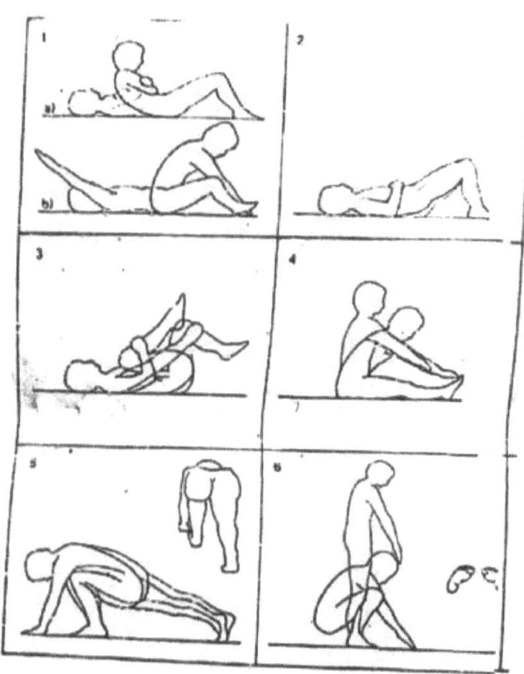

Bring your spine forward to touch tip of your toes. This exercise has the function of stretching the hamstrings muscles behind the legs as well.

5. This is an exercise to stretch the muscles in front of the pelvis. Begin this exercise by bending the left leg forward and extending the right leg back. Keeping the left foot on the floor, bend the left knee forward, feeling a stretch in the front of the right thigh. After repeating this ten times, flex the right leg forward and do the exercise with the other leg.

6. The last exercise is like sitting in an Indian closet. This is called the static squat.

   Most of these exercises are less comfortable for those who suffer from knee pain. William exercise is good to repeat three times daily for those without other ailments.

67. Now I have understood the William's exercises, along with the exercises mentioned at the beginning such as pelvic tilt, rowing and chin up. Now, can you elaborate on correcting the posture of the body?

Of course.

Correct body posture is important for standing, sitting and driving. The abnormal posture is one of the most easily correctable causes of back pain, Postural Defects requires knowledge of the changes in the spine during our development before birth in order to understand the correct Posture. At birth there is a single curve in the middle of the whole spine. Then, as a result of raising the head, cervical lordosis is gradually formed in the neck and, with standing, lumbar lordosis is formed behind the abdomen. Both these curves are considered part of the natural process. But depending on the lack or excess of these curves, neck pain and back pain are seen.

68. OK. But how do you know the grades of these curves that don't cause back pain?

That's what I'm going to explain. There is an easy way to find out this. Change the clothes so that the curves of the waist are visible to some extent. Then stand with your midsection against a wall with your feet 10 cm apart. In this position, the head, shoulders and back should be touching the wall. Then ask if the palm of the hand will cross in the middle behind the navel.

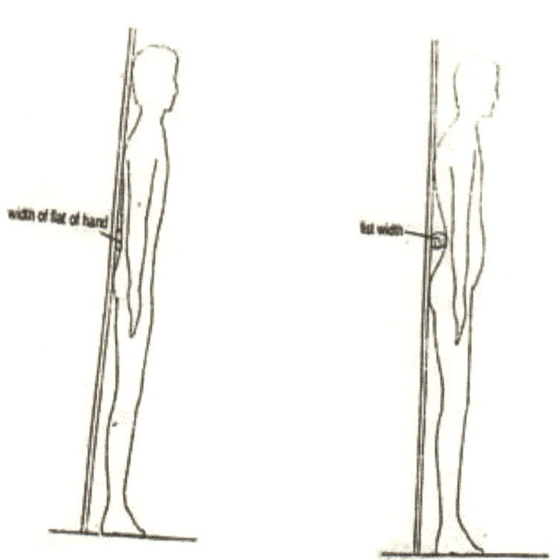

Lumbar lordosis can be assumed to be in the correct range if it is possible only by flat position of the palm. However, in a state of increased lordosis, the clenched fist can be passed.

69. What is work related back pain?

Certain jobs are more likely to cause back pain. For example, Nursing is a field where you have to bend forwards and backwards for patient care. Similarly, there are many jobs that require heavy lifting. Those who do jobs that involve pushing or pulling heavy objects also experience back pain. House maids, dentists, etc. are all prone to back pain. All this is called work related back pain.

70. What should be done to avoid work related back pain?

The main thing is to do things that require less strain on the mid-body, such as lifting weights, pushing and pulling.

For example, three guidelines are given when weight lifting.

1. Stand as close as possible to the weight to be lifted. Foot should be 45 cm apart. One foot behind the weight to be lifted and the second leg should be slightly to the side of it.

2. Then bend next to a heavy object with knees bent. Hold the weight with both hands so that the waist does not bend.

3. Lift weight close to our body without bending the elbows and take with the strength of the leg muscles. This is will reduce the strain on back.

71. Often when going to an orthopaedic OP with back pain, the doctor examines and writes a diagnosis of mechanical back pain on the ticket. What is mechanical back pain?

Very good question.

There are many causes of back pain. Depending on the location of the pain, it can be classified as neck pain, shoulder pain, mid back, and low back and coccygeal pain

But depending on the causes it can be classified as direct cause and indirect cause. 80% of these causes are caused by indirect causes. Direct causes of back pain include infections, tumors, tuberculosis, osteoporosis, spondylosis, fractures, and spondylolysis But the indirect, or avoidable causes are due to the defects in our life style with lot of mental and physical stress. Indirect causes of low back pain include poor postural habits, depression, improper lifting weight at work, non-routine strenuous work, and inappropriate work place habits. This is called mechanical back pain.

At the same time, in addition to 20% of the direct causes of back pain, problems like urinary tract disorders, gastrointestinal diseases, prolapsed uterus in women and other uterine diseases can also cause back pain. It is on the basis of this information that a doctor performs the necessary tests to make his diagnosis and arrive at the right treatment.

72. Is back pain a gender-specific disease?

Osteoporosis, coccygenea and piriformis syndrome, which cause back pain, are more common in women, but diseases such as ankylosing spondylitis are more common in men.

73. What is osteoporosis?

The name osteoporosis comes from the meaning of porous bones. It is a disease in which the bone density or bone mass decreases and consequently the structure of the bones weakens. Without proper treatment and care, sufferers of this disease get their bones broken due to minor injuries. This is called fragility fracture. This disease is more common in postmenopausal women. Osteoporosis is a major cause of bone fractures in their wrists, hips, and vertebrae. It occurs in one-third of women over the age of fifty. Bone mass in women decreases by up to 20% within six years after menopause. More women die of hip fractures and bedridden deaths from osteoporosis than from cancers of the female reproductive organs such as the uterus, ovaries, and cervix.

The awareness of this disease in the society is not so widespread. This is because bone loss occurs without any other symptoms. That's why this disease is known as silent killer.

74. Why is osteoporosis more common in women than in men?

Good question.

Maximum bone strength is seen between the ages of 20 and 30. This is called peak bone mass. After the age of thirty, bone mass decreases by half to one percent annually. This varies from person to person. But this bone loss increases at a higher rate in women around and after menopause. Studies show that one reason for this is hormonal changes in women. For example, the hormone estrogen decreases in women after menopause.

Because of this, osteoporosis is more common in women.

75. What are the other causes leading to osteoporosis?

Causes can be broadly classified into two, modifiable and non modifiable. Modifiable factors are, Low calcium intake, alcoholism, very thin body habitus, premature menopause or menopause before the age of 45, low estrogen hormone. Absence of menses for more than a year before menopause, sedentary lifestyle, lack of exercise, vitamin D deficiency etc.

But reasons like old age, female gender, tradition etc. are non modifiable. Apart from these, there are many secondary causes of bone loss also.

Gastroinfestinal diseases such as Crohn's disease and severe liver diseases are among them. Rheumatoid arthritis, ankylosing spondylitis, osteogenesis imperfecta, hematologic diseases like lymphoma, multiple myeloma, hemophilia, thalassemia, and endocrine diseases like hyperthyroidism and Cushing syndrome are secondary causes. If we know that people who suffer from these diseases also have osteoporosis, we can prevent the resulting fractures.

76. What are the symptoms of osteoporosis?

Back pain is not the only thing seen in patients with osteoporosis. Many patients report that their legs are cramping. Another symptom is bone pain, especially at night. Decreased height in women after menopause is a sign of osteoporosis Neck pain, aching bones, fatigue, brittle nails, and tooth loss are also symptoms of osteoporosis.

77. How is osteoporosis diagnosed?

Bone mineral density or BMD is mainly used to diagnose osteoporosis. Deca QCT or Quantitative CT Scan, Peripheral DEXA, Single Photon Absorptiometry (SPA), Single Energy X-ray Absorptiometry and Radiographic Absorptiometry are also used for diagnosis.

78. How is osteoporosis treated?

Eat more calcium and vitamin D. Regular exercise is also good. And the thing to watch out for is to prevent falls. It is also not good to reduce weight beyond a certain limit.

79. What are the exercises for osteoporosis?

It is good to engage in exercise and activities like walking, running, tennis and dancing from the childhood itself.

Resistance exercises are also good to a certain extent. These include calf raises, knee bends, hip extensions, hip flexions, lateral leg raises, leg raises, knee extensions, shoulder strengthening, triceps lift, biceps curl, etc.

80. Why the osteoporosis is called silent killer ?

That's a good question. We know that, a person with hypertension without proper treatment can lead to heart attacks. Similarly, people with osteoporosis tend to break bones in sites such as the wrist, hip, and spine. To avoid this, people who are prone to osteoporosis should take measures to protect the bones and strengthen the bones. But most people live without knowing this possibility and knowledge, resulting In fractures and become bedridden. Hence it is called silent killer.

81. How can osteoporosis be controlled by increasing bone strength?

Bone mass regulation also has some mechanism in the body, just as diabetic patients control the blood glucose level without fluctuation. It can be classified into four. First tis the factors those increase bone mass deposition. These are the things that accelerate the activity of osteoblasts, the bone-producing cells. Exercises like walking, running, and growth help it.

Second is factors that slow down bone mass deposition. Alcoholism, chronic malnutrition and aging are the reasons for this.

Third is the deceleration of cells known as osteoclasts that resorb bone mass. These include hormones like Estrogen, Testosterone and Calcitonin. Fourth is factors that accelerate bone mass resorption through increased activity of cells called osteoclasts.

Sedentary lifestyle, hyperthyroidism and other conditions like include lymphoma, myeloma, and hyperparathyroidism are the conditions that control the strength of the bones.

82. Is there any awareness program now about this silent killer ?

Yes, There is.

World Osteoporosis Day is observed on October 20 every year. In this regard, various awareness activities are conducted all over the world. Each year each topic related to this disease is chosen as the theme for that year. The programs are conducted with the aim of giving awareness to the people.

83. Can joint pain occur without arthritis?

One reason for that is piriformis syndrome. Sitting for long periods of time results in this condition.

Excessive climbing, walking long distance etc. can also cause this problem. Although such patients approach the doctor with hip pain, the actual cause is the shortening of the pyriforms muscle. Improper exercise methods, incorrect running style, femoral anti-version, forefoot varus etc. lead to this. Often spinal disorders such as disc protrusion and spinal stenosis lead to these problems.

84. How is a person diagnosed with pyriformis syndrome?

A study on this disease was first published in 1928 in the world-famous journal Lancet. The pyriformis muscle is one of six muscles known as lateral rotators that rotate the hip outward. The sciatic nerve, the main nerve to the legs, passes through or under this muscle. It is attached from the bottom of the spine to the top of the femur bone.

This disease is diagnosed mainly through symptoms and tests. Pain is felt when pressing on the center of the muscle. Moreover, the buttocks will feel burning pain. Pain is often reported in the buttock and the middle of the back, or sacrum. It increases when sitting and walking. It decreases when lying down. Lifting and rotating the hips back and forth can be painful. Then you will see weakness. Pain and numbness in the leg will be there where the sciatic nerve supplies sensation.

85. What are the tests to diagnose piriformis syndrome?

Other less obvious diseases such as disc prolapse were unknown in the population a hundred years ago. Until then, such sufferers were accused of superstitious belief that something had come in the guise of a demon. It is through detailed studies that the scientific world has understood the details of this disease. Lie on your side so that the painful hip is in the upper side. Bend the painful leg and knock it on the examination stable where patient is lying. The patient complains of pain in the buttock when the affected knee is raised from the table. This diseases is diagnosed through this test.

86. How is Pyriformis Syndrome treated?

Pyriformis syndrome is treated in three stages. First of all, immediately after the injury to this muscle, i.e. two to three days of rest, painkillers, rubbing with ice, and keeping the leg slightly elevated are the treatment options. In the next stage, if the patient is not pregnant, heat treatment such as diathermy, ultrasound, hydrotherapy and massage treatment can be done. Next is the rehabilitation phase. This is where the help of physiotherapist is mainly needed. Exercises that strengthen the internal rotator and lateral hamstrings, as well as the external rotators and semitendinosus muscles, are commonly performed.

Pyriformis stretching exercise is also taught to patients. Stretch the pyriformis by crossing the affected leg over the opposite thigh while sitting straight. Muscles can also be strengthened and stretched through other methods. A good physiotherapist under the direction of a physical medicine and rehabilitation specialist doctor can teach this to the patients.

87. You did not say that a scan is required for diagnosis of any of the ailments now. But when we go to the hospital with back pain, doctors will request to take that scan. Isn't this something mysterious about that, doctor?

Never.

That is a misunderstanding. Fibromyalgia, Pyriformis Syndrome, Osteoporosis, Work Related Back pain and psychosomatic disorders, can be detected by other tests without a scan. But a scan is essential to rule out some other common diseases. Because only after confirming the diagnosis, we can decide the right treatment. Some of them even require surgery. This is why MRI scan is recommended for many back pain cases. Some details are understood. For example, a patient who has experienced persistent back pain for up to six months with no apparent cause may be asked to undergo a scan.

Similarly, if the pain going to the leg does not improve after four to six weeks with usual treatments, an MRI scan should be done. Another reason is, if there are some dangerous symptoms accompanied by back pain or cramps, we have to evaluate with MRI scan. These dangerous symptoms are called Red Flag symptoms. Patient with low back pain should be assessed for, previous cancer, unexplained weight loss, immunosuppression, urinary tract infections, long-term use of steroid drugs, and intravenous drug use. Symptoms known as red flag signs include lower back pain that does not respond to standard treatments, fatal falls, trauma, or bone loss in the elderly, sudden bladder obstruction or urinary retention, involuntary bowel movements, numbness in the buttocks, and weakness in the legs.

And because it is expensive, the common man views doctors with suspicion if MRI scan is advised.

Now X-rays can be taken at a low cost in all government hospitals. In future, MRI will be available at affordable cost in all government hospitals. Bringing the scan facility in government hospitals will clear these doubts

88. So what are the diseases with back pain those require surgery?

Intervertebral disc prolapse, canal stenosis and spondylolistheis are the main causes of back pain requiring surgery, other than spinal cord injury with vertebral bone fracture.

89. In short, back pain results from both trivial and serious causes. But some require surgery. Will you please tell symptoms which are to be evaluated carefully to rule out surgery in such illnesses ?

That's right. There are many causes of back pain. However, 70% of back pain resolves within two weeks without any major treatment. Ninety percent of back pain resolves within six weeks. In only 5% of cases, there are reasons that require surgery. It is in that category that one needs to pay more attention. There are some simple ways to do that.

First, try to lift the big toe up. If it doesn't work, it is assumed that the nerves coming from the spine to the legs may have been compressed. This is usually due to disc displacement. Then try to lift the other toes in the same way. If not, you should immediately consult an orthopedic specialist for advice. Similarly, another simple test is to check for touch sensation in the foot, toes, and leg with a cotton swab.

If the touch sensation is affected, further tests are required. Another thing to test is those who have difficulty in urination and bowel habits and they should undergo further tests to ensure that there is no condition that requires surgery.

90. All doctors say that self-medication should not be done. But often in some remote places the services of a doctor are not readily available. Then it would be good if there were some self-treatments that could be done temporarily but without major risks. Or should it not be?

That's a good question. I have felt that too. I have been given the opportunity to treat patients in many parts of Kerala as part of government job. For example, in many places in Alappuzha, the only transportation facilities are waterways. Similarly in districts like Kasaragod, Idukki and Wayanad there are many people living in hilly areas. In my experience, almost every district has places where there is a delay in getting expert treatment. It is a feature of our geographical variations. From time to time some things have changed due to improvements in government systems but not completely. So it is good to know some methods like first aid as a temporary relief.

First of all, as I said earlier, make sure that there are no serious diseases or illnesses that require any immediate medical treatment. After that, stay completely in bed for two days. This is called absolute bed rest. Then ice cold pack can be applied on the painful area.

Rubbing is good in the beginning. If the pain persists after two days, then it is better to apply heat. Then take pain killers only after consulting the nearest doctor. Do the exercises I mentioned earlier only if there is no pain. In addition follow the correct posture and correct method of weight lifting. Seek expert advice if necessary.

Belts, lumbosacral corsets, and bed rest with weighted traction should only be done under expert guidance.

91. Can back pain be cured by massaging ?

Many conditions, such as herniated discs and spondylolysis, do not change.

However, massage can help to reduce the pain and other side effects of many things. Chiropractic therapy can reduce muscle stiffness or spasm. Pain is relieved by reducing muscle spasm. As the pain decreases, so does the stiffness. Thus, massaging is useful. In addition, muscle in fibrotic tissue with fibrotic nodules known as trigger spots that cause long-term chronic pain can be removed by skilled massage or injection. Many causes of these fibrotic nodules have been identified. Many people can find similar nodules or lumps in many muscles behind our bodies around the spine. Studies show that 80% of people with this condition have a reduction in two weeks.

92. Can we do massage at home?

Massaging is a form of therapy. For that specific methods are suggested by the experts. This is done in several steps. Let's explain it a little.

Stretching or massaging is not effective for all causes of back pain. However, it has been found to be effective in treating conditions such as fibromyalgia. But it should be done in the right way. Otherwise, there are many patients who come complaining that the pain has increased ten fold after going for the massage.

Initially, lay the patient prone on a comfortable surface. After identification of the painful area, massage with a non-allergenic or non itchy oil from the shoulder joint downwards, bringing the fingertips closer to the center of the spine. Apply firm pressure to the finger tips and little finger area. When you reach the lower part of the waist, take the hands out and take them to the outer part of the buttock and return both the hands to the same place where they started. All this should be done in one movement without removing the hands from the patient's body. Similarly, during the downward movement, the body part of the masseur standing at the head side of the patient should be pressed with the force of the hands. Repeat this ten times.

As massage is a scientific method of treatment, it can be done with the help of an expert physiotherapist and is more effective if we obtain advice from PMR specialist doctor (Physiatrist). As mentioned earlier, the massage can be repeated from each side of the patient with the fingers of one hand on top of the other By moving the hands in a circular motion with sufficient force, this massaging continues in such a way that from the side of the small sacro-iliac joint on both sides of the spine, it takes five centimeters out through the crest of the pelvis and reaches up to the shoulder blade itself.

Then do the same on the opposite side. Repeat ten times. Meanwhile, the small lump like nodules seen in fibromyalgia should be felt on the fingers and massaging should be done effectively focusing on them.

Similarly, fibrotic nodules in the buttocks can be detected by massaging the little finger of the hand, starting one inch from the center and working outwards in a circular motion to the top of the thigh. Repeat this three times on both sides.

This technique is called partner massage. Treatment methods such as massage are usually performed by a skilled physiotherapist under the guidance of a physical medicine and rehabilitation specialist (Physiatist). But in case of emergency, elderly parents who are bedridden at home or close relatives who are unable to take them to physiotherapy, this massaging method is explained here only as a temporary measure for very close relatives. Partner massage should be completed by repeating only the first part of the above procedure. As mentioned above, stand at the head of the patient lying on his back and bring the fingers together and bring the hands down only and repeat ten times.

A massage can provide temporary relief for sudden back pain. Fibromyalgia can also be relieved to some extent by focused frictional massage on the outside of the fibrotic nodules.

93. What are the causes of neck pain?

There are many reasons. The causes of neck pain can be broadly classified into four. First and foremost is related to muscles. It can include the previously mentioned fibromyalgia and myofascial pain syndrome. Pain that spreads to the arm is called neuropathic pain. Pain from arthritis is caused by inflammation. There is also disc between the vertebrae of the neck. Just like back pain, a herniated disc can cause neck pain. This is called mechanical or compressive pain.

94. What are the causes of fibromyalgia?

This is mainly due to a decrease in the body's chemical known as serotonin, which is associated with our sleep and pain perception. This pain can be controlled to some extent by taking some available medicines. Some exercises like walking and swimming are good.

95. Massage therapy has been described earlier to treat myofascial trigger points. Other than this, what other treatment is there?

There are other medicines. Medications that reduce muscle spasms can be used. And then there is the injection. This is done by holding the nodules with two fingers and taking an injection. Treatment methods such as acupuncture are also used.

96. Can you explain about neuropathic pain?

It is a very unpleasant pain. Sufferers often describe it as burning or hooking. Often chronic musculoskeletal pain can later develop into neuropathic pain. It is common to see pain like this. Occurs due to entrapment of nerves or nerve roots.

97. How will you treat neuropathic pain?

First of all, the causes of pain should be removed. If muscle pain persists, evaluate for fibromyalgia or myofascial nodules and treat. If not, check if there are tumors or intervertebral disc prolapse that are trapping the nerves and take appropriate treatment. And if we talk about drug treatment, gel to apply on the painful area or painkillers are good. Also take other medicines like tricyclic antidepressants and baclofen only after prescribed by a doctor.

Then receive physical modality treatment such as TENS as prescribed by a physiatrist or physical medicine specialist.

98. What is TENS?

TENS or Transcutaneous Electric Nerve Stimulation is good for pain relief. It is a small machine that gives mild electrical stimulation to the painful area. Today it is available for self-administration by the patient. It works through gate control mechanism.

99. What is gate control mechanism?

This is called Melzack and Wall gate control theory. It would be better to explain it with a picture.

The pain stimulus travels along the C fibers of the nerve fibers. Fibers specialized for pain sensation reach the projection nerve in the spinal cord and thereby produce the sensation of pain in the brain. But when a mild electrical stimulus using TENS reaches the projection neuron via the A Beta fiber, the inhibitory interneuron is stimulated and it neutralizes the pain stimulus from the projection neuron to the brain.

Excitation of the projection neuron is inhibited by stimulation of the inhibitory interneuron. Thus the stimulus of pain to the brain disappears. The gate is closed. And the pain goes away. This is called the Melzack and Wall Gate Control Theory.

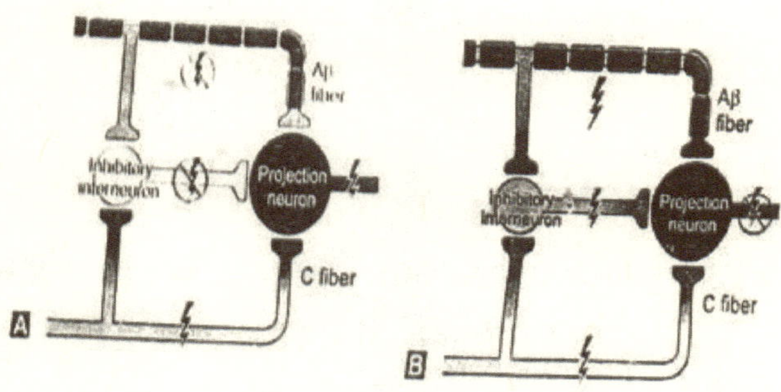

100. Why add Melzac and Wall to this?

This discovery was made by two scientists named Ronald Melzak and Patric Wall in 1965. Their gate control theory is known as one of the most influential studies on pain. This theory has made revolutionary progress in pain studies and research. That is why it is called the Melzack and Wall Gate Control Theory.

101. Where in the neck are the most common painful trigger points?

Good question.

Myofascial pain syndrome is a major cause of neck pain. Most Viewed In the trapezius muscle. In addition to the trapezius, trigger points or fibrotic nodules are also found in the levator scapula, infraspinatus, supraspinatus, suboccipital muscles, and anterior cervical muscles in front of the neck.